DENTAL HEALTH COOKBOOK FOR KIDS

Delicious Recipes to Promote Healthy Teeth and Gums for Kids!

SMART DESTY

Copyright © [2023], [Smart Desty]

All rights reserved. No part of this book may be reproduced, stored in a retrieval system, or transmitted in any form or by any means, electronic, mechanical, photocopying, recording, scanning, or otherwise, without the prior written permission of the copyright owner.

Table of Contents

Introduction

Dental health is an important part of overall health and nutrition. Our teeth are important for chewing and speaking, and they also play a role in the overall health of our bodies. Eating a nutritious and balanced diet is essential for maintaining good dental health, and it is important to ensure that children are getting all the necessary nutrients from their food.

This book is designed to help children and their parents learn about healthy eating habits and the importance of keeping teeth clean and healthy.

The Dental Health Cookbook for Kids will help parents and children learn about healthy eating habits and the importance of keeping teeth clean and healthy. The recipes in this book are all kid friendly, easy to make and delicious! From breakfast to dinner, snacks to desserts, and even tooth-friendly treats, this book has something for everyone.

In addition to providing recipes and tips to help kids learn how to make healthy food choices, this book also includes information on dental hygiene, how to properly care for teeth and gums, and the importance of visiting the dentist regularly. There are also activities and games to help kids learn more about dental health.

The Dental Health Cookbook for Kids is part of a larger effort to promote good oral health in children. It is important that children learn the importance of taking care of their teeth and how to make healthy food choices. This book is a great resource that can be used to help teach kids about the importance of taking care of their teeth, and to help parents provide healthy meals for their families.

The Dental Health Cookbook for Kids is filled with fun and educational recipes, activities, and information that will help kids learn about dental health. There are recipes for breakfast, lunch, dinner, snacks, and desserts that are all kid friendly and easy to make. The activities provided are designed to help kids learn more about dental health and to help parents provide healthy meals for their families.

The Dental Health Cookbook for Kids also includes information about oral hygiene, tips for proper care of teeth and gums, and information about the importance of regular visits to the dentist. This book is a great resource for parents and children alike, and can be used to help teach kids about dental health and to help parents provide healthy meals for their families.

We hope that this book will help parents and children learn more about dental health, and that it will help create a healthier and happier lifestyle for everyone. Thank you for taking the time to check out the Dental Health Cookbook for Kids!

Chapter 1:
Healthy Eating Habits

Good dental health is a critical part of overall health, and it starts in childhood. By teaching your children healthy eating habits, you can set them up for a lifetime of strong dental health.

The first step in teaching your children healthy eating habits is to limit their intake of sugary and acidic foods. These foods, such as candy, soda, and fruit juices, can cause tooth decay and erosion. Instead, focus on serving more nutrient-rich foods such as fresh fruits and vegetables, whole grains, lean proteins, and low-fat dairy products. Encourage them to drink plenty of water, which will help keep their teeth and mouth clean.

Next, establish a regular dental hygiene routine and make it fun. Let your kids pick out their own toothbrush and toothpaste and make sure they brush their teeth twice a day for two minutes each time. You can even set a timer and make it a game. Additionally, make sure your kids floss daily to remove any food particles that are stuck between their teeth.

It is pertinent for you as a parent or guidance to be a role model for your children. Demonstrate healthy eating habits and dental hygiene habits by leading by example. Make sure to schedule regular dental checkups for your children, so that any dental issues can be identified and addressed quickly.

These simple steps will help ensure that your children maintain good oral health. By teaching your kids healthy eating habits and establishing a regular dental hygiene routine, you can help them develop good oral hygiene habits that will last a lifetime.

Chapter 2:
Nutrition Basics

A nutritious diet is necessary for strong teeth and gums. Eating a balanced diet with plenty of fruits, vegetables, and whole grains is important for overall health, as well as dental health.

Consuming foods that are high in calcium and vitamin D are especially important for keeping teeth and gums healthy. Strong bones and teeth require calcium, and vitamin D facilitates the body's absorption of calcium. Dairy products, such as milk, cheese, and yogurt, are good sources of calcium and vitamin D. Other calcium-rich foods include almonds, spinach, and fortified cereals.

Fruits and vegetables are also important for dental health. Fruits and vegetables contain vitamins and minerals that help to keep teeth and gums healthy. They also provide fiber, which helps to clean the teeth and freshen breath.

It's also crucial to avoid eating too much sugar and carbs. Sugary snacks and drinks, such as candy and soda, can increase the risk of tooth decay. Starchy foods, such as bread and chips, can also contribute to tooth decay if not properly brushed and flossed away.

In addition to eating a balanced diet, practicing good oral hygiene is essential for dental health. Brushing twice a day with a fluoride toothpaste and flossing once a day can help to keep teeth and gums healthy. Regular visits to the dentist for cleanings and check-ups are also important.

Nutrition is an important part of overall health, and good nutrition is essential for healthy teeth and gums. Eating a balanced diet with plenty of fruits, vegetables, and whole grains, limiting sugary and starchy foods, and practicing good oral hygiene are all important for dental health.

Chapter 3:
Teeth-Friendly Recipes

Breakfast Recipes

Twenty (20) Dental Friendly Breakfast Recipes for Kids with prep time, calories and instructions.

1. Banana Oat Pancakes:

Prep Time: 10 minutes; Calories: 188; **Instructions**: Mash 1 ripe banana in a large bowl. Add 1 cup of oats, 1 tsp of baking powder, and 1 cup of milk and stir until combined. Heat a nonstick pan over medium heat and spray with cooking spray. Drop the batter into the pan, cook until bubbles form on the edges and flip. Cook till golden brown on low heat.

2. Baked Apple Oatmeal:

Prep Time: 10 minutes; Calories: 218; **Instructions**: Preheat oven to 350°F. Grease an 8x8 baking dish with non-stick cooking spray. In a medium bowl, combine 1 cup of rolled oats, 1 cup of almond milk, 2 tablespoons of maple syrup, 1 teaspoon of cinnamon, 1 teaspoon of vanilla extract, 1 teaspoon of baking powder, and a pinch of salt. Mix until combined. Add in 1 diced apple and mix again. Pour mixture into the greased baking dish. Bake for 25-30 minutes, until golden brown and cooked through.

3. Greek Yogurt Parfait:

Prep Time: 5 minutes; Calories: 190; **Instructions**: Layer ½ cup of Greek yogurt with ¼ cup of granola and ¼ cup of fresh berries in a bowl or parfait cup. Top with a drizzle of honey and a sprinkle of cinnamon.

4. Egg and Avocado Toast: Prep Time: 10 minutes; Calories: 250.

Instructions: Toast two slices of whole wheat bread. In a small bowl, whisk together 1 egg and 1 tablespoon of milk. Heat a nonstick pan over medium heat and spray with cooking spray. Pour egg mixture into the pan and cook until set. Spread mashed avocado onto the toast and top with the cooked egg. Add salt and pepper according to taste.

5. Banana and Almond Butter Smoothie:

Prep Time: 5 minutes; Calories: 235; **Instructions**: Place 1 banana, 1/2 cup of almond milk, 1 tablespoon of almond butter, 1 teaspoon of honey, and a few ice cubes into a blender. Blend until smooth.

6. Berry and Greek Yogurt Breakfast Bowl: Prep Time: 5 minutes; Calories: 148; **Instructions**: Top ½ cup of Greek yogurt with ½ cup of fresh berries, 1 tablespoon of sliced almonds, and 1 teaspoon of honey.

7. Whole Wheat Waffles:

Prep Time: 10 minutes; Calories: 200; **Instructions**: In a medium bowl, mix together 1 cup of whole wheat flour, 1 teaspoon of baking powder, 1 teaspoon of sugar, and a pinch of salt. In a separate bowl, whisk together 1 cup of milk, 1 egg, and 1 tablespoon of melted butter. Pour the wet ingredients into the dry ingredients and whisk until combined. Heat a waffle iron to medium heat and spray with cooking spray. Cook the batter in the waffle maker until it turns golden.

8. Overnight Oats: Prep Time: 5 minutes; Calories: 219.

Instructions: In a medium bowl, combine 1/2 cup of rolled oats, 1/2 cup of almond milk, 1 tablespoon of chia seeds, 1 tablespoon of maple syrup, 1 teaspoon of cinnamon, and a pinch of salt. Mix until combined. Overnight, cover and place in the refrigerator. In the morning, top with fresh fruit and nuts.

9. Chocolate Peanut Butter Oatmeal: Prep Time: 5 minutes; Calories: 313; **Instructions**: In a medium saucepan, bring 1 cup of almond milk to a gentle boil. Add 1/2 cup of oats, 1 tablespoon of cocoa powder, 1 tablespoon of peanut butter, 1 teaspoon of honey, and a pinch of salt. Stir until combined. Simmer for five minutes over low heat, stirring occasionally.Serve and top with fresh fruit and nuts.

10. Baked Oatmeal Cups:

Prep Time: 10 minutes; Calories: 176; **Instructions**: Preheat oven to 375°F. Use cooking spray that is non-stick to grease a muffin pan. In a medium bowl, mix together 1 cup of rolled oats, ¼ cup of maple syrup, 1 teaspoon of baking powder, and a pinch of salt. Add 1 cup of almond milk and mix until combined. Evenly divide the oat mixture between the muffin tin cups. Until golden brown, bake for 15 minutes.

11. Savory Egg and Cheese Sandwich: Prep Time: 10 minutes; Calories: 335; **Instructions**: Heat a nonstick pan over medium heat and spray with cooking spray. Crack 2 eggs into the pan and cook until set. Place the eggs on top of one slice of whole wheat bread, top with 1 slice of cheese, and the other slice of bread.

12. Greek Yogurt and Fruit Bowl: Prep Time: 5 minutes; Calories: 224; Instructions: Top ½ cup of Greek yogurt with ½ cup of fresh fruit, 1 tablespoon of slivered almonds, and 1 teaspoon of honey.

13. Blueberry Muffins:

Prep Time: 10 minutes; Calories: 140; **Instructions**: Preheat oven to 350°F. Use nonstick cooking spray to coat a 12-cup muffin pan. In a medium bowl, mix together 1 cup of whole wheat flour, 1 teaspoon of baking powder, 1 teaspoon of cinnamon, and a pinch of salt. In a separate bowl, whisk together 1 cup of milk, 1 egg, 1 tablespoon of melted butter, and 1/4 cup of honey. Combine the dry ingredients with the wet components after adding them. Fold in 1 cup of fresh blueberries. Divide the batter among the muffin cups in an even amount. Bake for 20 minutes, until golden brown.

14. French Toast Sticks:

Prep Time: 10 minutes; Calories: 156; **Instructions**: In a shallow dish, whisk together 2 eggs, 1 tablespoon of milk, 1 teaspoon of cinnamon, and a pinch of salt. Dip 4 slices of whole wheat bread into the egg mixture, making sure to coat both sides. Heat a nonstick pan over medium heat and spray with cooking spray. Slices of bread should be cooked in the pan until golden brown. Cut into sticks and serve with fresh fruit.

15. Fruit and Nut Bars: Prep Time: 10 minutes; Calories: 248;

Instructions: Preheat oven to 350°F. Use nonstick cooking spray to grease an 8x8 baking dish. In a medium bowl, mix together 1 cup of rolled oats, 1/2 cup of almond flour, 1/4 cup of sliced almonds, 1/4 cup of honey, 1 teaspoon of cinnamon, 1/4 teaspoon of salt, and 1/4 cup of melted butter. Press the mixture into the greased baking dish. Bake for 15 minutes, until golden brown. Let cool and cut into bars.

16. Egg and Cheese Bagel Sandwich: Prep Time: 10 minutes; Calories: 383; **Instructions**: Toast one whole wheat bagel. Spray cooking spray into a nonstick pan and heat it up over medium heat.Crack 2 eggs into the pan and cook until set. Place the eggs on top of one half of the bagel, top with 1 slice of cheese, and the other half of the bagel.

17. Peanut Butter and Banana Toast:

Prep Time: 5 minutes; Calories: 250; **Instructions**: Toast two slices of whole wheat bread. Spread 1 tablespoon of peanut butter onto each slice and top with sliced banana.

18. Oatmeal and Banana Bites:

Prep Time: 10 minutes; Calories: 196; **Instructions**: Preheat oven to 350°F. Grease a 12-cup mini muffin tin with non-stick cooking spray. In a medium bowl, mix together 1 cup of rolled oats, 1/4 cup of melted butter, 1/4 cup of honey, 1 teaspoon of cinnamon, and a pinch of salt. Place 1 teaspoon of the oat mixture into each mini muffin cup and press down to form a cup.

Bake for 10 minutes. Let cool and top each cup with a sliced banana.

19. Apple Cinnamon Muffins:

Prep Time: 10 minutes; Calories: 160; **Instructions**: Preheat oven to 350°F. Use nonstick cooking spray to coat a 12-cup muffin pan. In a medium bowl, mix together 1 cup of whole wheat flour, 1 teaspoon of baking powder, 1 teaspoon of cinnamon, and a pinch of salt. In a separate bowl, whisk together 1 cup of almond milk, 1 egg, 1 tablespoon of melted butter, and 1/4 cup of honey. Combine the dry ingredients with the wet components after adding them. Fold in 1 diced apple. Until golden brown, bake for 20 minutes.

20. Chocolate Chia Seed Pudding:

Prep Time: 5 minutes; Calories: 179; **Instructions**: In a medium bowl, mix together 1/2 cup of chia seeds, 1/2 cup of almond milk, 1 tablespoon of cocoa powder, 1 tablespoon of maple syrup, and a pinch of salt. Stir until combined. Add fresh fruit and nuts to the top in the morning.

Lunch Recipes

Twenty (20) Dental Friendly Lunch Recipes for Kids with prep time, calories and instructions.

1. Peanut Butter and Banana Toast:

Prep time: 5 minutes. Calories: 250. **Instructions**: Spread a tablespoon of peanut butter onto 2 slices of whole grain toast. Place a sliced banana on top of the peanut butter and serve.

2. Mediterranean Yogurt Bowl:

Prep time: 5 minutes. Calories: 320. **Instructions**: Place ½ cup of plain Greek yogurt in a bowl. Top with ½ cup of sliced cucumbers, ¼ cup of diced tomatoes, and ¼ cup of chopped kalamata olives. Sprinkle with oregano and sea salt.

3. Vegetable Tostadas:

Prep time: 10 minutes. Calories: 200. **Instructions**: Spread a tablespoon of refried beans on each tostada shell. Top with some shredded lettuce, diced tomatoes, and shredded cheese. Place on a baking sheet and bake for 8 minutes at 350°F.

4. Turkey Roll-Ups: Prep time: 5 minutes. Calories: 200.

Instructions: Take two slices of deli turkey and spread a tablespoon of cream cheese on each slice. Place a few slices of cucumbers or tomatoes in the center and roll up.

5. Egg Salad Sandwich:

Prep time: 10 minutes. Calories: 300. **Instructions**: Hard boil two eggs and mash with a fork. Stir in a tablespoon of mayonnaise, a teaspoon of mustard, and a pinch of salt and pepper. Spread the egg salad on two slices of bread and serve.

6. Veggie Wrap: Prep time: 10 minutes. Calories: 250.

Instructions: Spread a tablespoon of hummus on a whole wheat wrap. Top with lettuce, diced tomatoes, and sliced cucumbers. Roll up and cut in half.

7. Avocado and Cheese Quesadilla:

Prep time: 10 minutes. Calories: 300. **Instructions**: Spread a tablespoon of mashed avocado on a whole wheat tortilla. Sprinkle with shredded cheese and top with another tortilla. Cook in a pan for a few minutes until cheese is melted.

8. Turkey and Cheese Pita Pockets:

Prep time: 10 minutes. Calories: 330. **Instructions**: Place two slices of deli turkey and two slices of cheese in a pita pocket. Add lettuce and diced tomatoes and serve.

9. Apple and Peanut Butter Bites:

Prep time: 5 minutes. Calories: 250. **Instructions**: Spread a tablespoon of peanut butter onto a slice of apple. Sprinkle with some cinnamon and cut into slices.

10. Broccoli and Cheddar Baked Potatoes: Prep time: 10 minutes. Calories: 350. **Instructions**: Bake two potatoes in the oven at 400°F for 45 minutes. Top with steamed broccoli and shredded cheese and bake for another 10 minutes.

11. Fruit and Yogurt Parfait:

Prep time: 5 minutes. Calories: 250. **Instructions**: Layer ½ cup of plain Greek yogurt with ½ cup of fresh fruit such as blueberries and strawberries. Top with a sprinkle of granola for crunch.

12. Apple and Cheddar Bites:

Prep time: 5 minutes. Calories: 250. **Instructions**: Cut an apple into slices and top each slice with a thin slice of cheddar cheese.

13. Veggie and Hummus Pinwheels:

Prep time: 10 minutes. Calories: 200. **Instructions**: Spread a tablespoon of hummus on a whole wheat tortilla. Top with diced vegetables such as peppers, onions, and tomatoes. Roll up and cut in half.

14. Baked Chicken Nuggets:

Prep time: 10 minutes. Calories: 250. **Instructions**: Cut two chicken breasts into small chunks and place on a baking sheet. Sprinkle with garlic powder, paprika, and salt. Bake for 10 minutes at 375°F.

15. Baked Potato Fries:

Prep time: 10 minutes. Calories: 200. **Instructions**: Cut two potatoes into thin strips and place on a baking sheet. Sprinkle with olive oil, garlic powder, and salt. Bake for 15 minutes at 400°F.

16. Ants on a Log: Prep time: 5 minutes. Calories: 150.

Instructions: Spread a tablespoon of peanut butter onto celery sticks. Place some raisins on top and serve.

17. Carrot and Hummus Snack:

Prep time: 5 minutes. Calories: 150. **Instructions**: Slice up some carrots and serve with a side of hummus for dipping.

18. Cucumber and Cream Cheese Bagel Bites: Prep time: 10 minutes. Calories: 300. **Instructions**: Spread a tablespoon of cream cheese on a mini bagel. Top with a few slices of cucumber and bake for 8 minutes at 350°F.

19. Tuna Salad Sandwich:

Prep time: 10 minutes. Calories: 300. **Instructions**: Mix a can of tuna with a tablespoon of mayonnaise and a teaspoon of mustard. Spread some of the tuna salad onto two slices of bread and serve.

20. Baked Zucchini Chips:

Prep time: 10 minutes. Calories: 300. **Instructions**: Cut two zucchinis into thin slices and place on a baking sheet. Salt and olive oil should be drizzled on top. Bake for 15 minutes at 400°F.

Dinner Recipes

Twenty(20) Dental Friendly Dinner Recipes for Kids with prep time, calories and instructions.

1. Baked Chicken Fingers with Sweet Potato Fries: Prep Time: 10 minutes; Calories: 590;

Instructions: Preheat oven to 425 degrees F. Combine 2 cups breadcrumbs, 1 teaspoon garlic powder, 1/4 teaspoon black pepper, and 1/4 teaspoon salt in a shallow bowl. Dip 4 chicken breasts into beaten egg and then into the breadcrumb mixture. Chicken should be put on a baking sheet with parchment paper. Bake for 12 minutes, flipping halfway through. While the chicken bakes, cut 2 sweet potatoes into wedges and place on a baking sheet lined with parchment paper. Bake for 12 minutes, flipping halfway through. Serve chicken fingers with sweet potato fries.

2. Salmon and Broccoli Stir Fry:

Prep Time: 10 minutes; Calories: 368; **Instructions**: Heat 1 tablespoon olive oil in a skillet over medium-high heat. Add 2 cloves of minced garlic and cook for 1 minute. Add 2 cups fresh broccoli florets and cook for 3 minutes or until tender. Move the broccoli to one side of the skillet and add 8 ounces of salmon fillets. Cook for 3-4 minutes per side or until cooked through. Add a pinch of salt and pepper and stir in 1/4 cup of low-sodium soy sauce. Serve.

3. Turkey and Cheese Quesadillas:

Prep Time: 10 minutes; Calories: 441; **Instructions**: Heat a skillet over medium-high heat. Place 2 whole-wheat tortillas in the skillet and top with 1/2 cup shredded turkey, 1/2 cup shredded cheese, and 1/2 cup diced bell peppers. Allow to cook for 3 minutes or until golden brown. Flip the quesadilla over and cook for an additional 3 minutes. Cut into triangles and serve with your favorite salsa.

4. Zucchini Noodle and Meatballs:

Prep Time: 20 minutes; Calories: 334; **Instructions**: Heat 1 tablespoon olive oil in a skillet over medium-high heat. Add 1/2 cup diced onion and cook for 3 minutes. Add 1 pound ground turkey and cook for 8 minutes or until cooked through. Add 1 teaspoon garlic powder, 1 teaspoon Italian seasoning, and a pinch of salt and pepper. Stir in 1/2 cup marinara sauce. In a separate skillet, heat 1 tablespoon olive oil over medium-high heat. Add 2 zucchini spiraled into noodles and cook for 2 minutes. Add the cooked meatballs and marinara sauce to the skillet with the zucchini noodles and cook for an additional 2 minutes. Serve.

5. Baked Sweet Potato Fries and Veggie Nuggets:

Prep Time: 20 minutes; Calories: 565; **Instructions**: Preheat oven to 425 degrees F. Cut 2 sweet potatoes into wedges and place on a baking sheet lined with parchment paper. Bake for 15 minutes, flipping halfway through. While the potatoes bake, prepare the veggie nuggets. In a bowl, combine 1 cup shredded carrots, 1/4 cup diced onion, 1/4 cup diced celery, 1/4 cup diced bell pepper, 1 teaspoon garlic powder, 1 teaspoon Italian seasoning, and 1/4 teaspoon black pepper. Form the mixture into 4 nuggets and place on a baking sheet lined with parchment paper. Until golden brown or Bake for 12 minutes. Serve sweet potato fries with veggie nuggets.

6. Grilled Cheese and Tomato Soup: Prep Time: 10 minutes; Calories: 441; **Instructions**: Heat 1 tablespoon olive oil in a skillet over medium-high heat. Place 2 slices of whole-wheat bread in the skillet and top with 1/4 cup shredded cheese. 3 minutes of cooking time or until golden brown. Flip the grilled cheese over and cook for an additional 3 minutes. Meanwhile, heat 1/2 cup low-sodium tomato soup in a small pot. Serve grilled cheese with tomato soup.

7. Cheesy Baked Ziti:

Prep Time: 20 minutes; Calories: 590; **Instructions**: Preheat oven to 350 degrees F. Heat 1 tablespoon olive oil in a skillet over medium-high heat. Add 2 cloves of minced garlic and cook for 1 minute. Add 1/2 cup diced onion and cook for 3 minutes. Add 1/2 cup diced bell pepper and cook for an additional 3 minutes. Stir in 1 cup marinara sauce and simmer for 5 minutes. In a large pot, bring 4 cups of water to a boil. Add 8 ounces of ziti pasta and cook for 8 minutes or until al dente. Pasta that has been drained should be combined with marinara. Stir in 1/2 cup shredded cheese and 1/4 cup grated Parmesan cheese. Pour the ziti into a baking dish and top with 1/2 cup shredded cheese. 15 minutes of baking or until cheese is melted and bubbly.

8. Turkey Taco Bowls:

Prep Time: 10 minutes; Calories: 514; **Instructions**: Heat 1 tablespoon olive oil in a skillet over medium-high heat. Add 1/2 pound ground turkey and cook for 8 minutes or until cooked through. Add 1 teaspoon taco seasoning, 1 teaspoon garlic powder, and 1/4 teaspoon black pepper. Stir in 1/2 cup salsa. Divide the turkey mixture among 4 bowls. Top with 1/4 cup diced tomatoes, 1/4 cup shredded cheese, 1/4 cup shredded lettuce, and 1/4 cup diced avocado. Serve.

9. Baked Tilapia with Asparagus:

Prep Time: 20 minutes; Calories: 220; **Instructions**: Preheat oven to 400 degrees F. Place 4 tilapia fillets on a baking sheet lined with parchment paper. Top with 1 tablespoon olive oil, 1 teaspoon garlic powder, and a pinch of salt and pepper. Bake it for 12 minutes or until cooked through. Meanwhile, heat 1 tablespoon olive oil in a skillet over medium-high heat. Add 1/2 pound asparagus and cook for 5 minutes or until tender. Serve tilapia with asparagus.

10. Macaroni and Cheese with Broccoli:

Prep Time: 20 minutes; Calories: 551; **Instructions**: Bring 4 cups of water to a boil in a large pot. Add 8 ounces of elbow macaroni and cook for 8 minutes or until al dente. Pasta should be drained and added back to the saucepan.Stir in 1/2 cup shredded cheese and 1/4 cup grated Parmesan cheese. In a skillet over medium-high heat, heat 1 tablespoon olive oil. Add 1/2 cup broccoli florets and cook for 3 minutes or until tender. Add the broccoli to the macaroni and cheese and stir until combined. Serve.

11. Baked Egg Rolls with Rice:

Prep Time: 20 minutes; Calories: 484; **Instructions**: Preheat oven to 375 degrees F. In a bowl, combine 2 cups cooked white rice, 1/2 cup shredded carrots, 1/2 cup diced bell pepper, 1/2 cup diced onion, 1/4 cup diced mushrooms, 1 teaspoon garlic powder, and 1 teaspoon sesame oil. Place the mixture onto a baking sheet lined with parchment paper. Form into 8 egg rolls and bake for 15 minutes or until golden brown. Serve with your favorite dipping sauce.

12. Fish Sticks with Mashed Potatoes:
Prep Time: 20 minutes; Calories: 614;
Instructions: Preheat oven to 425 degrees F. Place 4 fish fillets onto a baking sheet lined with parchment paper. Top with 1 tablespoon olive oil and a pinch of salt and pepper. Bake it for 12 minutes or until cooked through. Meanwhile, peel and cut 2 potatoes into cubes. Boil in a pot of water for 10 minutes or until tender. Drain the potatoes and mash with 1 tablespoon butter, 1/4 cup milk, and a pinch of salt and pepper. Serve fish sticks with mashed potatoes.

13. Turkey Burger Sliders with Sweet Potato Fries:

Prep Time: 20 minutes; Calories: 515;
Instructions: Preheat oven to 425 degrees F. In a skillet set over medium-high heat, warm 1

tablespoon of olive oil. Add 1/2 pound ground turkey and cook for 8 minutes or until cooked through. Form into 4 sliders and cook for 3 minutes per side or until golden brown. Cut 2 sweet potatoes into wedges and place on a baking sheet lined with parchment paper. Bake for 15 minutes, flipping halfway through. Serve sliders with sweet potato fries.

14. Black Bean Burritos:

Prep Time: 10 minutes; Calories: 628; **Instructions**: In a skillet set over medium-high heat, warm 1 tablespoon of olive oil. Add 1/2 cup diced onion and cook for 3 minutes. Add 1 cup black beans, 1 teaspoon garlic powder, and 1/4 teaspoon black pepper. Cook beans for five minutes, or until heated thoroughly. Place the bean mixture onto 4 whole-wheat tortillas and top with 1/4 cup shredded cheese. Roll up the burritos and serve with your favorite salsa.

15. Peanut Butter and Banana Smoothie:

Prep Time: 10 minutes; Calories: 456; **Instructions**: Place 1/2 cup milk, 1/2 banana, 1 tablespoon peanut butter, 1 tablespoon honey, and 1/2 teaspoon vanilla extract into a blender. Blend until smooth. Serve.

16. Chicken Noodle Soup:

Prep Time: 20 minutes; Calories: 439; **Instructions**: Heat 1 tablespoon olive oil in a large pot over medium-high heat. Add 1/2 cup diced onion and cook for 3 minutes. Add 1/2 cup diced carrots, 1/2 cup diced celery, 1 teaspoon garlic powder, 1 teaspoon Italian seasoning, and a pinch of salt and pepper. Cook for an additional 5 minutes. Add 4 cups chicken broth and bring to a boil. Add 8 ounces of egg noodles and cook for 8 minutes or until al dente. Add 1/2 pound cooked chicken and simmer for 5 minutes. Serve.

17. Spaghetti and Meatballs:

Prep Time: 20 minutes; Calories: 654; **Instructions**: Bring 4 cups of water to a boil in a large pot. Add 8 ounces of spaghetti and cook for 8 minutes or until al dente. In a skillet, heat 1 tablespoon olive oil over medium-high heat. Add 1/2 pound ground beef and cook for 8 minutes or until cooked through. Add 1 teaspoon garlic powder, 1 teaspoon Italian seasoning, and a pinch of salt and pepper. Form the meat into 4 meatballs and add to the skillet. Cook for an additional 5 minutes. the pasta should be drained and return to the pot. Stir in 1 cup marinara sauce and the cooked meatballs. Serve.

18. Baked Tofu with Veggies:

Prep Time: 20 minutes; Calories: 431; **Instructions**: Preheat oven to 375 degrees F. Cut 1 package of extra-firm tofu into cubes. On a baking sheet covered with parchment paper, spread out the cubes. Top with 1 tablespoon olive oil, 1 teaspoon garlic powder, 1 teaspoon sesame oil, and a pinch of salt and pepper. 15 minutes baking time or until golden brown. One tablespoon of olive oil is heated over medium-high heat in a skillet. Add 1/2 cup diced onion and cook for 3 minutes. Add 1/2 cup diced bell pepper and cook for an additional 3 minutes. Serve baked tofu with veggies.

19. Chicken and Broccoli Alfredo:

Prep Time: 20 minutes; Calories: 590; **Instructions**: Bring 4 cups of water to a boil in a large pot. Add 8 ounces of fettuccine and cook for 8 minutes or until al dente. Return the spaghetti to the saucepan after draining it. Heat 1 tablespoon olive oil in a skillet over medium-high heat. Add 2 cloves of minced garlic and cook for 1 minute. Add 1/2 pound cooked chicken and cook for 5 minutes or until heated through. Add 1/2 cup broccoli florets and cook for an additional 3 minutes. Stir in 1/2 cup Alfredo sauce and simmer for 5 minutes. Pour the sauce over the pasta and stir until combined. Serve.

20. Baked Apple Oatmeal:

Prep Time: 10 minutes; Calories: 441; **Instructions**: Preheat oven to 350 degrees F. In a bowl, combine 1/2 cup rolled oats, 1/4 cup diced apple, 1 teaspoon ground cinnamon, 1 tablespoon honey, and 1/2 cup milk. Pour into a baking dish and top with 1/4 cup shredded coconut. Bake for 15 minutes or until golden brown. Serve with a dollop of yogurt.

Snack Recipes

Ten (10) Dental Friendly Snack Recipes for Kids with prep time, calories and instructions

1. Apple Slices with Peanut Butter

(Prep time: 5 minutes, Calories: 197): Slice an apple into thin pieces and spread a tablespoon of peanut butter on each slice. Enjoy!

2. Oatmeal with Berries

(Prep time: 5 minutes, Calories: 216): Cook 1/2 cup of oats in a pot of boiling water. Once the oats are cooked, mix in a handful of fresh or frozen berries. Enjoy!

3. Yogurt Parfait

(Prep time: 5 minutes, Calories: 164): Layer 1/2 cup of yogurt with a handful of fresh or frozen berries, a tablespoon of chia seeds, and a tablespoon of granola. Enjoy!

4. Banana with Nut Butter

(Prep time: 5 minutes, Calories: 130): Spread a tablespoon of nut butter onto a banana. Enjoy!

5. Carrot Sticks with Hummus

(Prep time: 5 minutes, Calories: 90): Cut one carrot into thin sticks and dip them into a tablespoon of hummus. Enjoy!

6. Celery with Cream Cheese

(Prep time: 5 minutes, Calories: 64): Spread a tablespoon of cream cheese onto celery sticks. Enjoy!

7. Apple with Cheddar Cheese

(Prep time: 5 minutes, Calories: 227): Slice an apple into thin pieces and top with a slice of cheddar cheese. Enjoy!

8. Cranberry Trail Mix

(Prep time: 10 minutes, Calories: 530): Mix together 1/2 cup of roasted almonds, 1/4 cup of dried cranberries, 1/4 cup of dark chocolate chips, and 1/4 cup of sunflower seeds. Enjoy!

9. Cheese and Crackers

(Prep time: 5 minutes, Calories: 261): Place a slice of cheese onto a cracker. Enjoy!

10. Kale Chips

(Prep time: 10 minutes, Calories: 110): Preheat oven to 375 degrees. Toss 1/2 cup of kale in 1 tablespoon of olive oil, 1 tablespoon of nutritional yeast, and a pinch of salt. Spread evenly on a baking sheet and bake for 10 minutes. Enjoy!

Chapter 4:
Beverages and Smoothies

Fifteen (15) Dental Friendly Beverages and Smoothies Recipes for Kids with prep time, calories and instructions

1. Banana-Mango Smoothie

– Prep Time: 5 minutes | Calories: 130

Instructions: Place 1 cup of diced mango, 1 frozen banana, and 1/2 cup of low-fat yogurt in a blender and blend until smooth.

2. Blueberry-Yogurt Smoothie

Preparation Time: 5 minutes | Calories: 120

Instructions: Place 1/2 cup of blueberries, 1/2 cup of low-fat yogurt, 1/2 cup of orange juice, and 1 teaspoon of honey in a blender and blend until smooth.

3. Strawberry-Banana Smoothie

– Prep Time: 5 minutes | Calories: 180

Instructions: Place 1/2 cup of sliced strawberries, 1 frozen banana, 1/2 cup of low-fat yogurt, and 1 tablespoon of honey in a blender and blend until smooth.

4. Apple-Cinnamon Smoothie

– Prep Time: 5 minutes | Calories: 150

Instructions: Place 1/2 cup of diced apples, 1/2 cup of low-fat yogurt, 1/2 cup of apple juice, 1 teaspoon of cinnamon, and 1 tablespoon of honey in a blender and blend until smooth.

5. Blueberry-Oat Smoothie

– Prep Time: 5 minutes | Calories: 160

Instructions: Place 1/2 cup of blueberries, 1/4 cup of oats, 1/2 cup of low-fat yogurt, and 1/2 cup of almond milk in a blender and blend until smooth.

6. Pineapple-Coconut Smoothie

– Prep Time: 5 minutes | Calories: 150

Instructions: Place 1 cup of diced pineapple, 1/2 cup of low-fat yogurt, 1/4 cup of coconut milk, and 1 teaspoon of honey in a blender and blend until smooth.

7. Orange-Carrot Smoothie

– Prep Time: 5 minutes | Calories: 140

Instructions: Place 1/2 cup of grated carrots, 1/2 cup of orange juice, 1/2 cup of low-fat yogurt, 1 teaspoon of honey, and a pinch of cinnamon in a blender and blend until smooth.

8. Avocado-Spinach Smoothie

Preparation Time: 5 minutes | Calories: 120

Instructions: Place 1/2 cup of spinach, 1/2 of a ripe avocado, 1/2 cup of low-fat yogurt, and 1 tablespoon of honey in a blender and blend until smooth.

9. Banana-Berry Smoothie

– Prep Time: 5 minutes | Calories: 150

Instructions: Place 1/2 cup of mixed berries, 1 frozen banana, 1/2 cup of low-fat yogurt, and 1 tablespoon of honey in a blender and blend until smooth.

10. Peach-Yogurt Smoothie

– Prep Time: 5 minutes | Calories: 140

Instructions: Place 1/2 cup of diced peaches, 1/2 cup of low-fat yogurt, 1/2 cup of almond milk, and 1 tablespoon of honey in a blender and blend until smooth.

11. Mango-Kiwi Smoothie

– Prep Time: 5 minutes | Calories: 130

Instructions: Place 1 cup of diced mango, 1 kiwi, and 1/2 cup of low-fat yogurt in a blender and blend until smooth.

12. Cherry-Almond Smoothie

– Prep Time: 5 minutes | Calories: 160

Instructions: Place 1/2 cup of pitted cherries, 1/2 cup of low-fat yogurt, 1/4 cup of almond milk, 1 teaspoon of honey, and 1 teaspoon of almond extract in a blender and blend until smooth.

13. Banana-Cocoa Smoothie

– Prep Time: 5 minutes | Calories: 140

Instructions: Place 1 frozen banana, 1/2 cup of low-fat yogurt, 1/4 cup of almond milk, 1 tablespoon of cocoa powder, and 1 teaspoon of honey in a blender and blend until smooth.

14. Papaya-Ginger Smoothie

Preparation Time: 5 minutes | Calories: 120

Instructions: Place 1 cup of diced papaya, 1/2 cup of low-fat yogurt, 1/2 teaspoon of grated ginger, and 1 tablespoon of honey in a blender and blend until smooth.

15. Apple-Cinnamon Smoothie

Preparation Time: 5 minutes | Calories: 120

Instructions: Place 1/2 cup of diced apples, 1/2 cup of low-fat yogurt, 1/4 cup of almond milk, 1 teaspoon of cinnamon, and 1 tablespoon of honey in a blender and blend until smooth.

Chapter 5:

Dental-Friendly Desserts

Ten (10) Dental Friendly Desserts Recipes for Kids with prep time, calories and instructions

1. Baked Apples: Prep time: 10 minutes; Calories: 190;

Instructions: Preheat your oven to 350 degrees F. Cut the top off of each apple and use a spoon to scoop out the insides, creating a hollow center. Fill the hollow of each apple with a tablespoon of brown sugar, a teaspoon of butter, and a sprinkle of cinnamon. Bake the apples for 10 minutes or until the apples are soft and the sugar is melted.

2. Protein Pudding: Prep time: 5 minutes; Calories: 130;

Instructions: Mix 2 scoops of protein powder with 1 cup of non-fat milk in a bowl, stirring until the powder is fully dissolved. Divide the mixture among 4 small containers and refrigerate for 1 hour until it has set. Enjoy!

3. Banana Ice Cream:

Prep time: 5 minutes; Calories: 50; **Instructions**: Peel and slice 3 ripe bananas. Place the slices in a zip-top bag and freeze for at least 2 hours. Once frozen, blend the slices in a food processor or blender until smooth. Serve immediately.

4. Yogurt Parfait: Prep time: 5 minutes; Calories: 160;

Instructions: Layer 1 cup of plain yogurt with 1/4 cup of granola and 1/2 cup of fresh berries in a bowl. Drizzle with honey if desired. Enjoy!

5. Fruit Salad: Prep time: 10 minutes; Calories: 100;

Instructions: Combine 1 cup of diced pineapple, 1 cup of diced apples, 1/2 cup of diced mango, and 1/2 cup of diced kiwi in a bowl. Drizzle with 2 tablespoons of honey and 1 tablespoon of lemon juice. Enjoy!

6. Chocolate Banana Bites:

Prep time: 10 minutes; Calories: 80; **Instructions**: Peel and slice 2 ripe bananas.

Place the slices in a zip-top bag and freeze for at least 2 hours. Once frozen, dip the slices in melted dark chocolate and place them on a parchment-lined baking sheet. Freeze for another 2 hours. Enjoy!

7. Peanut Butter Energy Balls:

Prep time: 10 minutes; Calories: 135; **Instructions**: Place 1 cup of rolled oats, 1/2 cup of peanut butter, 1/4 cup of honey, and 1/4 cup of mini chocolate chips in a bowl. Mix until combined. Roll the mixture into 1-inch balls and keep refrigerated in an airtight container. Enjoy!

8. Chocolate-Dipped Strawberries:

Prep time: 10 minutes; Calories: 100; **Instructions**: Wash and dry 1 pint of fresh strawberries. Melt 1/2 cup of dark chocolate chips in the microwave in 30-second intervals, stirring in between until completely melted. Dip the strawberries in the melted chocolate and place them on a parchment-lined baking sheet. Refrigerate until firm. Enjoy!

9. Frozen Grapes: Prep time: 10 minutes; Calories: 40;

Instructions: Wash and dry 2 cups of fresh grapes. Place the grapes in a zip-top bag and freeze for at least 2 hours. Enjoy!

10. Apple Pie Smoothie:

Prep time: 5 minutes; Calories: 130;
Instructions: Place 1/2 cup of non-fat milk, 1/2 cup of plain yogurt, 1/2 of a peeled and cored apple, 1/4 teaspoon of ground cinnamon, and 1 tablespoon of honey in a blender. Blend until smooth. Serve immediately.

Chapter 5:

Dental Care Tips

Dental Care tips for kids:

1. Brush your teeth twice a day for two minutes each time. Use a soft-bristled toothbrush and fluoride toothpaste.

2. Floss your teeth every day to remove plaque and food particles that are stuck between your teeth.

3. Limit sugary snacks and drinks, as they can cause cavities.

4. Visit the dentist every six months for a professional cleaning and checkup.

5. If needed, use a mouthwash to help reduce plaque and freshen breath.

6. Use a fluoridated toothpaste and consider getting a fluoride treatment from your dentist to help strengthen your teeth.

7. Don't forget to brush your tongue! On your tongue, bacteria can accumulate and lead to bad breath.

8. If your child wears braces, make sure to brush and floss carefully around the wires and brackets.

9. Consider using sealants on your child's teeth as a way to protect them from cavities.

10. Set a good example for your child by brushing and flossing your own teeth every day.

11. Make sure your child wears a mouthguard while playing contact sports. This will help protect their teeth from injuries.

Chapter 6:
Making Dental Visits Fun

Making dental visits fun for kids can be a challenge, but it is an important part of helping them to develop good oral health habits. By taking the time to make each visit a positive experience, you can help to ensure that your child develops a lifetime of healthy teeth and gums.

One of the best ways to make dental visits fun for kids is to create a positive atmosphere. Make sure that the staff is friendly and welcoming, and that the waiting room has plenty of games and activities for kids to enjoy. This will help to make the experience of visiting the dentist a positive one.

Another way to make dental visits fun is to involve the child in the process. Ask them questions about their teeth and gums, and explain what the dentist is doing in simple terms. This will help them to feel more comfortable and understand what is happening.

It is also important to use incentives to make dental visits fun. For example, you can offer rewards for brushing and flossing every day. You can also offer small prizes such as stickers or candy after each visit. This will help to make the experience more enjoyable and encourage your child to practice good oral hygiene.

Finally, it is important to be patient and understanding when it comes to making dental visits fun for kids. It is normal for children to feel anxious or scared before going to the dentist, so it is important to be understanding and supportive. If they do become overwhelmed, take some time to talk to them and reassure them that there is nothing to be afraid of.

Overall, making dental visits fun for kids can be challenging, but it is essential for helping them to develop good oral health habits. By taking the time to create a positive atmosphere, involve the child in the process, and use incentives, you can help to ensure that each visit is a fun and enjoyable experience.

Conclusion

A dental health cookbook for kids is an invaluable resource for children to learn about healthy eating habits, proper oral care, and the importance of maintaining good dental health. It is especially useful for parents who want to help their children avoid cavities, gum disease, and other potential dental issues. The cookbook can help children develop a foundation of healthy eating habits, while also teaching them the importance of brushing and flossing regularly.

The cookbook contains recipes specifically designed to promote dental health in children. Many of the recipes include ingredients that are rich in calcium and other minerals, which are essential for healthy teeth and gums. Additionally, the recipes are designed to be easy for children to make, so parents can have confidence that their children will enjoy making them.

The cookbook also contains information about proper oral hygiene, such as how to brush, floss, and use mouthwash. It also provides guidance on the best type of toothpaste, toothbrush, and other dental products to use. Additionally, the cookbook can help parents teach their children the importance of visiting their dentist regularly for check-ups and cleanings.

In conclusion, the dental health cookbook for kids is an essential tool for parents who want to help their children develop healthy eating habits and maintain good oral hygiene. The recipes in the cookbook can help children learn to make nutritious meals, while also teaching them the importance of brushing and flossing regularly. Additionally, the book provides information on proper oral hygiene and the best dental products to use. Finally, the cookbook can help parents ensure their children are visiting their dentist regularly for check-ups and cleanings.

www.ingramcontent.com/pod-product-compliance
Lightning Source LLC
Chambersburg PA
CBHW061604250726
48657CB00017B/1866